AF228944

DEALING WITH ADDICTION

GAMING ADDICTION

by Kizzi Roberts

BrightPoint Press

San Diego, CA

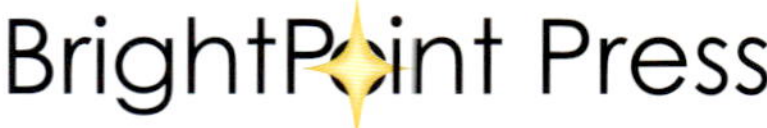

© 2023 BrightPoint Press
an imprint of ReferencePoint Press, Inc.
Printed in the United States

For more information, contact:
BrightPoint Press
PO Box 27779
San Diego, CA 92198
www.BrightPointPress.com

Content Consultant: Douglas Gentile, PhD, Professor of Psychology, Iowa State University

LIBRARY OF CONGRESS CATALOGING-IN-PUBLICATION DATA

Names: Roberts, Kizzi, 1987- author.
Title: Gaming addiction / by Kizzi Roberts.
Description: San Diego, CA: BrightPoint Press [2023] | Series: Dealing
   with addiction | Includes bibliographical references and index. |
   Audience: Grades 10-12
Identifiers: LCCN 2022008613 (print) | LCCN 2022008614 (eBook) | ISBN
   9781678203764 (hardcover) | ISBN 9781678203771 (eBook)
Subjects: LCSH: Video game addiction--Juvenile literature.
Classification: LCC RC569.5.V53 R64 2023 (print) | LCC RC569.5.V53
   (eBook) | DDC 616.85/84--dc23/eng/20220316
LC record available at https://lccn.loc.gov/2022008613
LC eBook record available at https://lccn.loc.gov/2022008614

CONTENTS

AT A GLANCE

- Gaming addiction is the dysfunctional use of video games.

- Estimating the number of people with gaming addiction is difficult. Researchers think between 1 and 10 percent of gamers become addicted.

- Young men are most likely to become addicted to gaming.

- Gaming addiction negatively affects a player's life. Its effects may include fatigue, depression, anxiety, anger, loss of relationships, and damage to physical health.

- The World Health Organization recognized gaming addiction as a disorder in 2018.

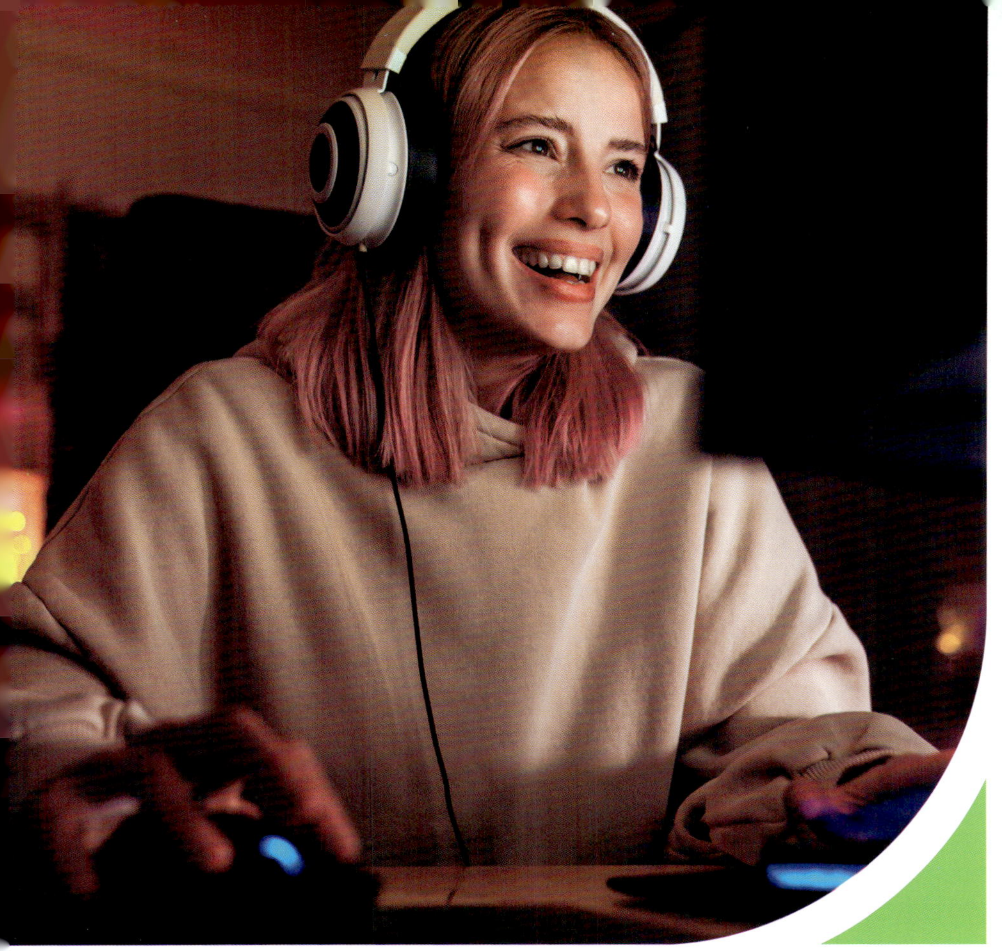

- Treatment options for gaming addiction include self-help, group therapy, and one-on-one therapy. Cognitive behavioral therapy can be an effective treatment for gaming addiction, too.

- Researchers continue to study gaming addiction.

CAN PLAYING GAMES BECOME A PROBLEM?

Ben loved playing video games. He played games before school and after school. On the weekends, Ben would play all day.

When his friends came over, Ben only wanted to play video games. His friends liked to play with him. But they liked doing

other things, too.

"Let's play baseball at the park," his

friend Carmen said.

"I'm beating my high score," Ben replied.

When his friends left, he did not even

say goodbye.

Playing video games with friends can be fun.

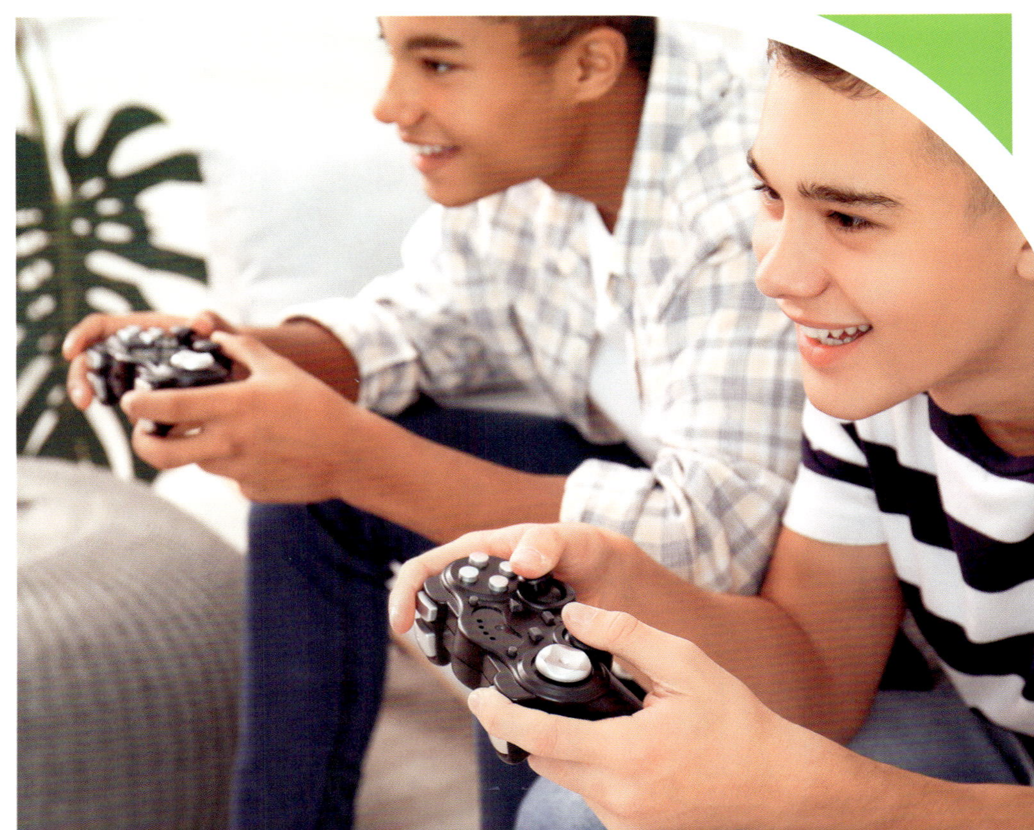

Ben missed out on time with his family, too. He did not eat dinner with them. Instead, he ate junk food in his room.

He stayed up late playing games. This made him tired at school. Ben often fell asleep in his first class. He would forget to do his homework. He failed tests because he forgot to study.

"Hey, sleepyhead," Carmen said as she shook him awake at lunch one Monday.

"Go away," Ben grumbled.

"Did you stay up all night playing games?"

"Not *all* night," Ben replied angrily.

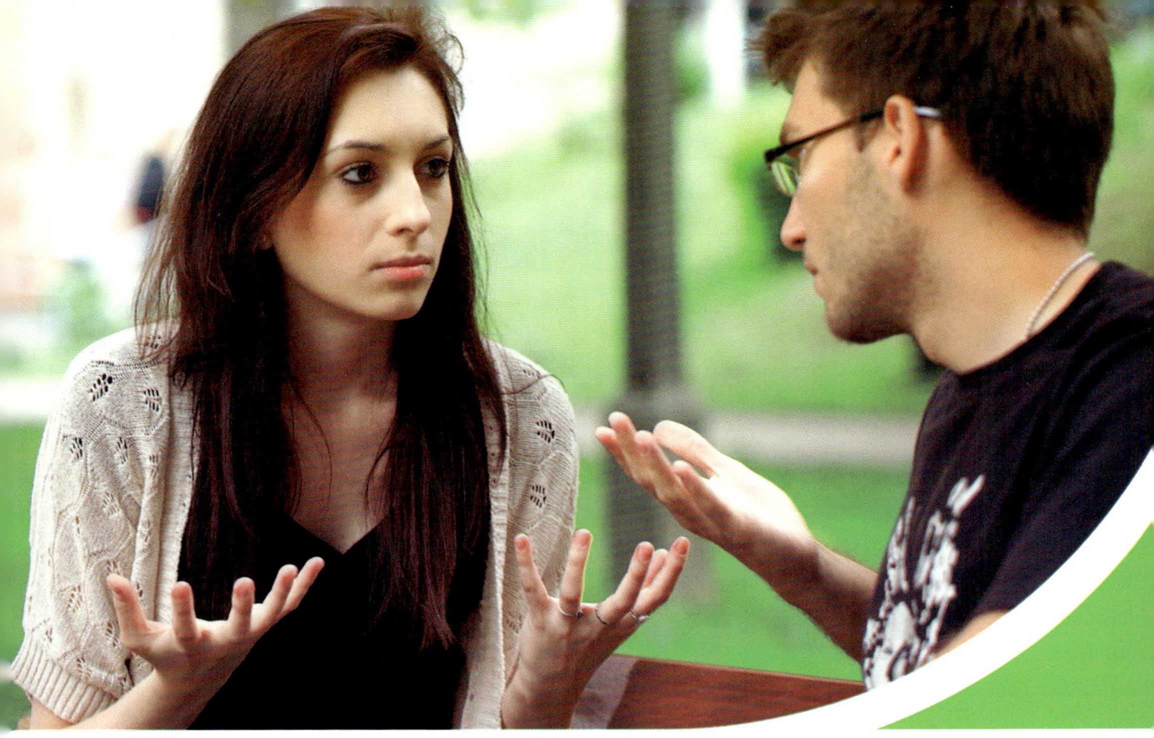

"I've been reading about gaming addiction," said Carmen. "I think you're addicted to video games. You play constantly. You never have time for anything else. You are tired all the time and behind in your classes. Sometimes you are angry, too."

Ben sighed. He said, "You might be right. I think I might have a problem. What should I do?"

Once Ben realized he might be addicted to video games, he could talk about it. He told his friends, his parents, and the school counselor about his problem. With help, Ben learned to balance his time between school, family, friends, and video games. Ben's health and relationships improved. He spent more time doing non-gaming activities he enjoyed.

Playing video games alone or with friends is fun. Not everyone who plays video games

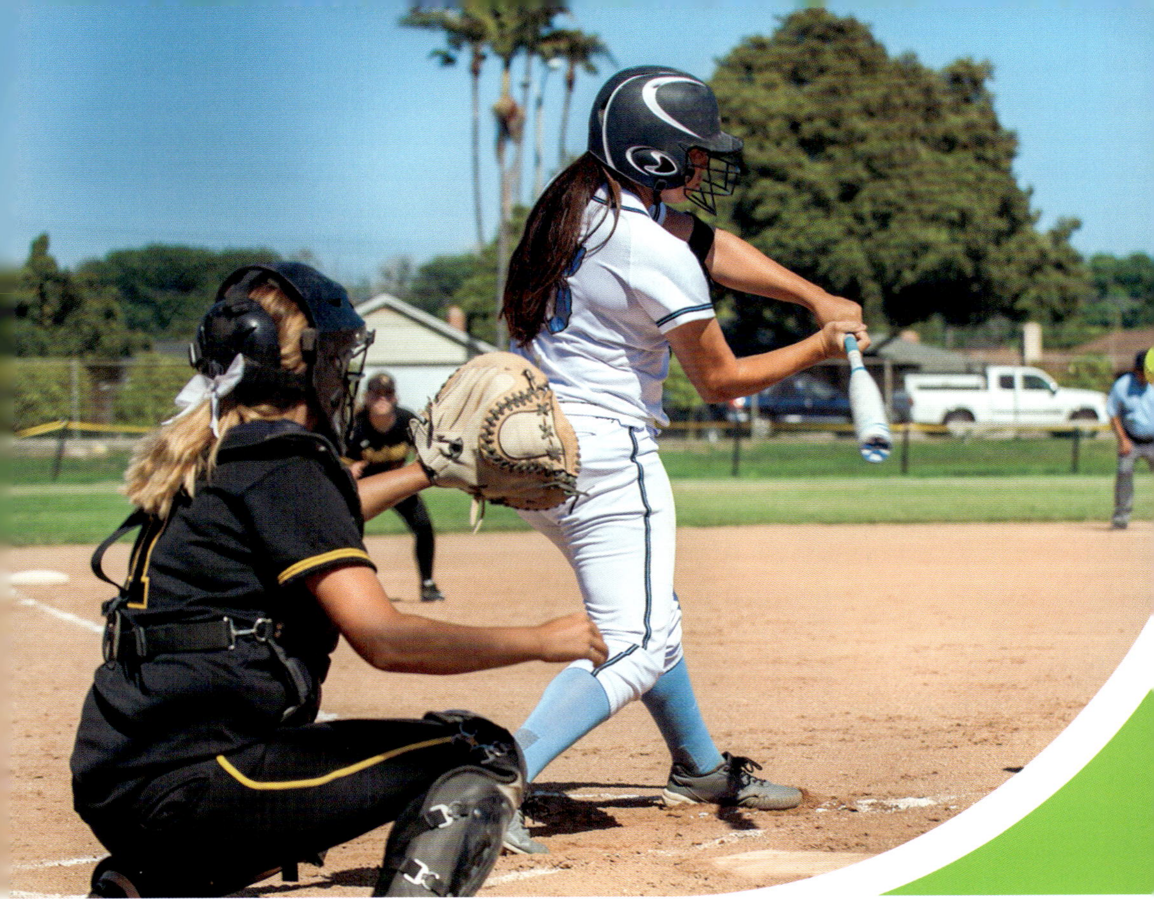

will become addicted. But some people

might. That is why it is important to know

the signs of addiction. Knowing the signs

helps people see a problem, get help, and

recover from an addiction.

1

WHAT IS GAMING ADDICTION?

People all over the world enjoy playing video games. People play games on consoles, computers, and handheld devices. Video games are very easy to access. This can cause some people to spend too much time playing. Time spent playing is not the only sign of trouble.

People will also **neglect** other important things to play video games. This can be a sign of a problem.

In 2018, the World Health Organization (WHO) recognized gaming addiction as a disorder. The WHO is an international

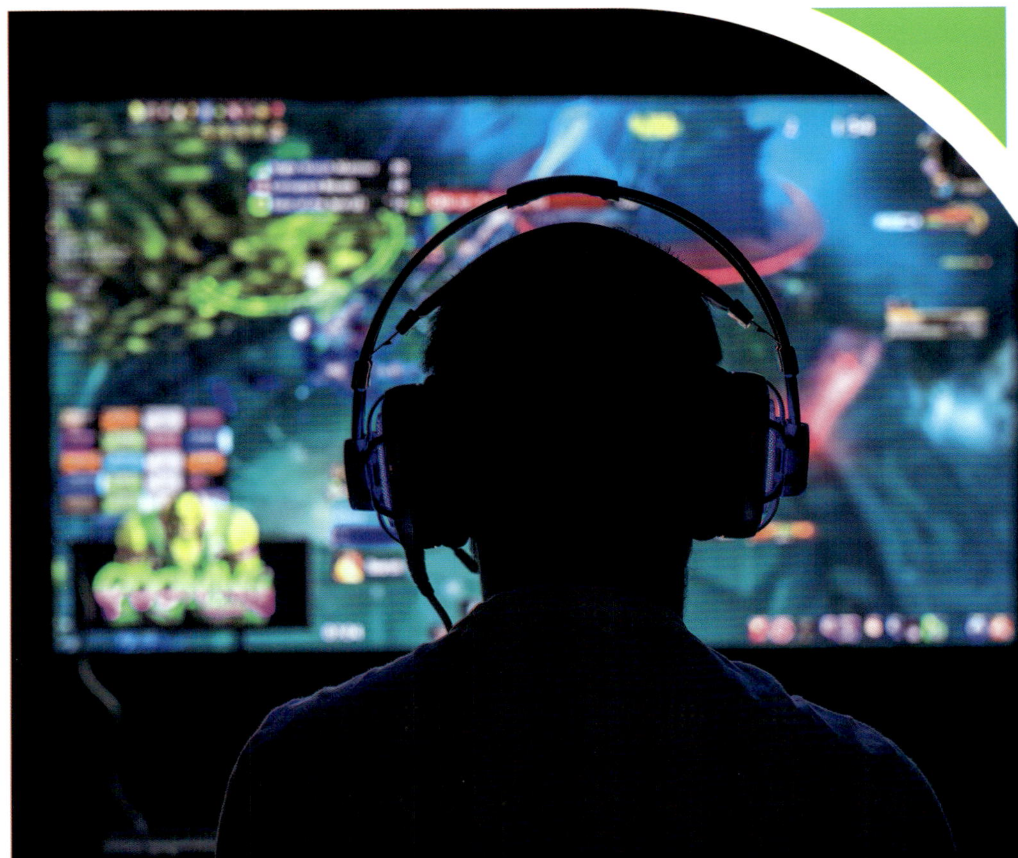

organization. It helps people around the world lead healthy lives. It uses scientific research to identify diseases and disorders.

The WHO defines several signs of gaming addiction. Someone may struggle to control the time he or she spends gaming. A person may prioritize "gaming over other activities to the extent that gaming takes precedence over other interests and daily activities."[1] Someone may continue to play despite **negative consequences**. Gaming may interfere with school or work.

The negative consequences of video game addiction can disrupt a person's life.

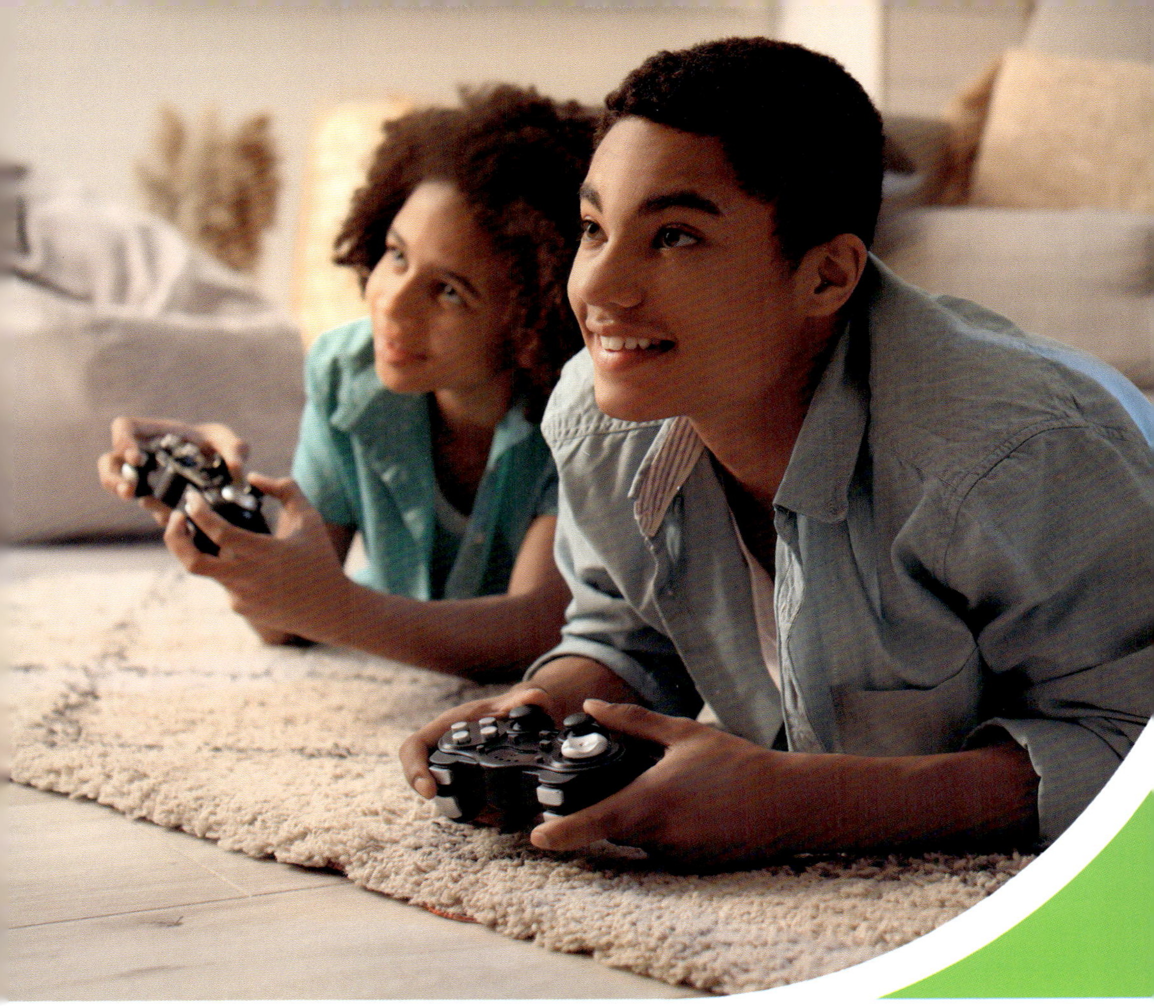

Gaming addiction affects the lives of a

player's friends and family, too. Therefore,

it is important to understand how gaming

addiction starts.

HOW DOES GAMING ADDICTION START?

People play video games for many reasons. Most people play because it is fun. Other people play to keep their brains active. Many games involve problem-solving and puzzles. People play video games to relax, too. Stanley Pierre-Louis is the president

GOT GAME?

In 2021, 76 percent of American kids aged eighteen and younger played video games. Of these gamers, 77 percent played with friends online or in person. Additionally, 74 percent of parents played video games with their children at least once a week.

and CEO of the Entertainment Software Association. According to Pierre-Louis, "Games transcend age, race, gender, platform and even political parties. Indeed, this is the United States of Play."[2]

Around the world, more than 3 billion people play video games. In 2020, at least one person played video games in 75 percent of US homes. Video games can be fun to play alone or with family and friends. More than three-quarters of all gamers play with other people. Many gamers make friends playing games.

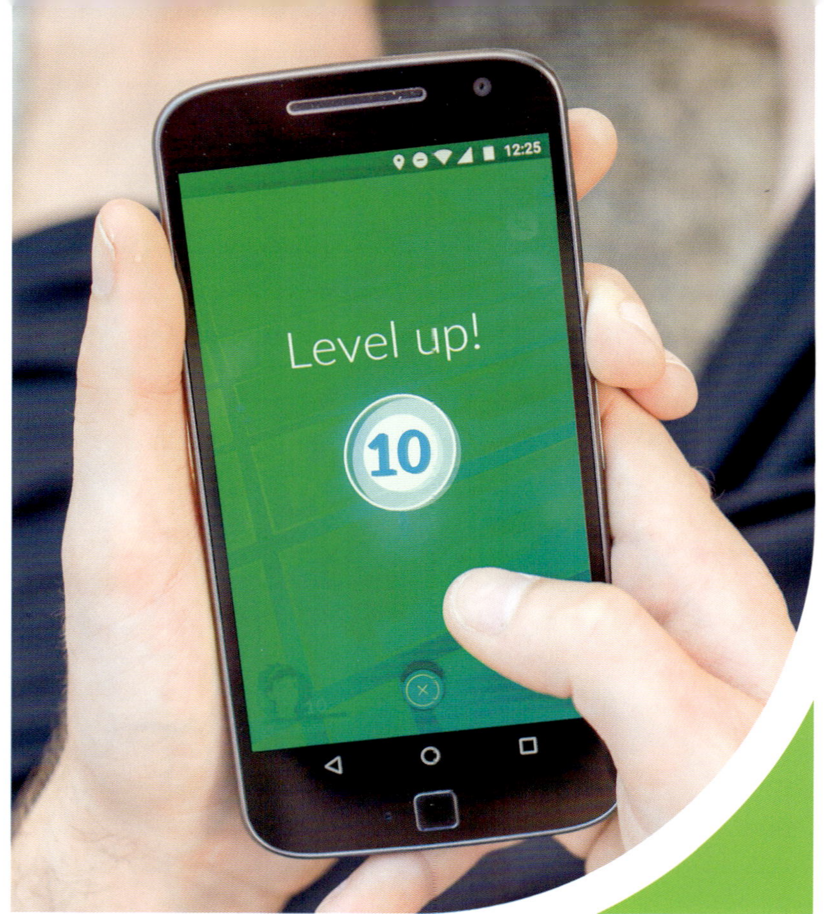

Leveling is one way game designers encourage people to keep playing.

These can be real-life friends. Other friends might be people they meet in-game.

Video games are designed to make sure the players are constantly having fun. Some games have different levels. Others have goals to unlock. People can make progress in the game and improve their skills.

However, playing video games can become a problem for some players. This can happen when someone spends so much time gaming that he or she neglects other important things. People can play games almost anywhere on smartphones, tablets, and handheld consoles. Many players game on computers and consoles. With many ways to play, it is easy for someone to play games all the time.

It is hard for people with gaming addiction to spend less time playing.

Gaming addiction makes people only want to play video games. Some people play video games and stop doing other activities. People with gaming addiction might get angry if they cannot play games. They might yell or become violent toward belongings or people. They might also get sad or anxious.

WHO IS MOST LIKELY TO BECOME ADDICTED TO VIDEO GAMES?

In 2016, Oxford University's Internet Institute surveyed nearly 19,000 gamers. The gamers lived in Germany, the United States, Canada, and the United Kingdom. The study found that up to 1 percent might suffer from gaming addiction. The next year, Japanese researchers looked at data gathered from many studies. Some studies found that gaming disorder affected less than 1 percent of the Japanese population. Others said it affected more than 25 percent of the population. The wide-ranging results show how hard it can be to identify people with gaming addiction. The exact number of players who become addicted to video games is unknown. Researchers estimate between 1 and 10 percent of gamers become addicted.

Anyone can become addicted to gaming. However, some people are more likely to become addicted than others. Experts believe men represent 83 percent of people addicted to gaming. Young men in their late teens and early twenties are most at risk of gaming addiction. However, young men in this age range are not the only people who

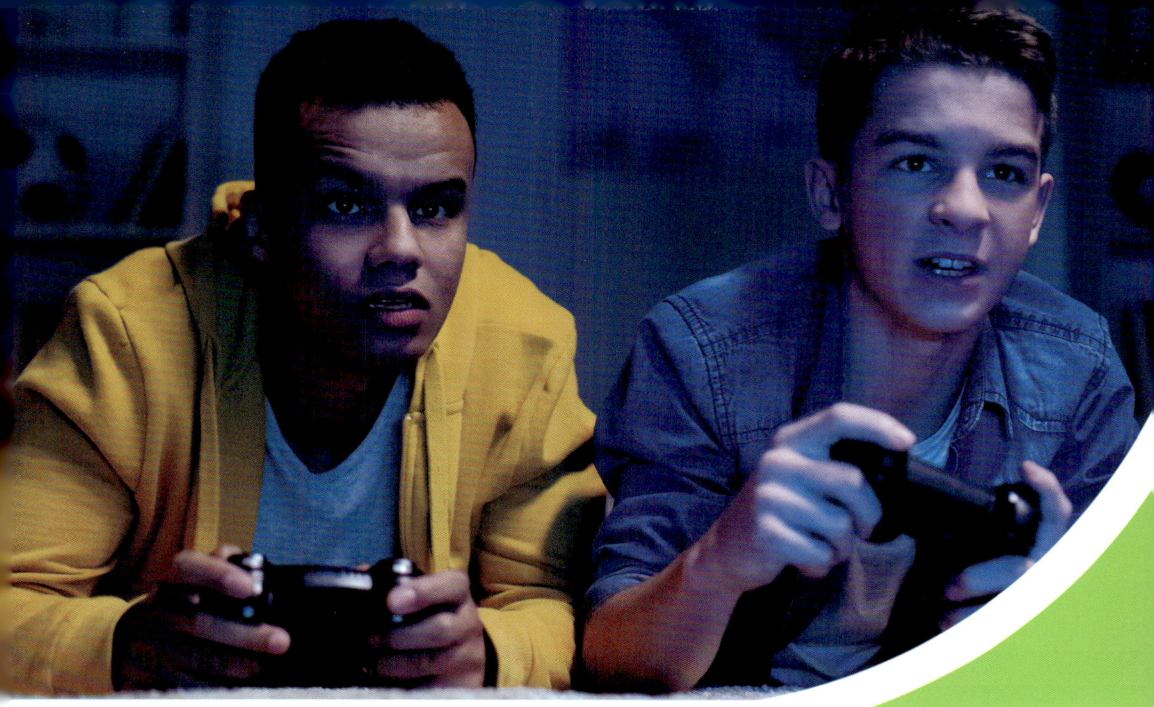

become addicted. They are simply more at

risk of addiction than other groups.

Not everyone who plays video games will

become addicted. Only a small percentage

of people who play video games develop

a problem. Most people have fun playing

video games without becoming addicted.

2
THE SCIENCE OF GAMING ADDICTION

Addiction is a **chronic** brain disease. It affects how the brain processes rewards, motivation, and memory. Addiction causes someone to obsessively use a substance or repeat a behavior. The person will do so even if it causes him or her harm. People with a history of addiction in their families are more likely to develop an addiction themselves.

Some people become addicted to alcohol or other drugs. Others become addicted to behaviors. They may obsessively gamble. Or they may play video

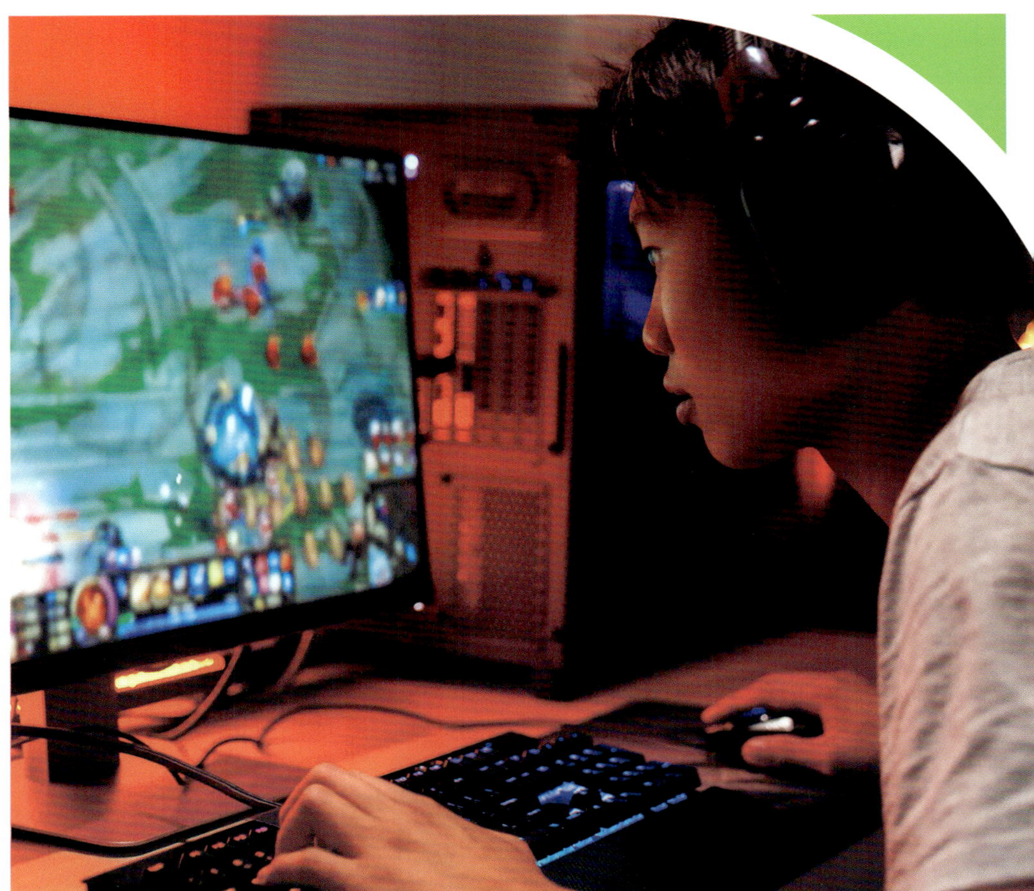

Obsessive gaming may be a sign of addiction.

games, even when doing so affects their grades, health, and relationships. Like other brain diseases, addiction can be treated. It can also be prevented.

The American Psychiatric Association (APA) supports research and education about mental disorders and mental health. In 2013, the APA recognized internet gaming disorder (IGD) as an emerging problem. It identified nine different symptoms of gaming addiction. These included being preoccupied with gaming and experiencing unpleasant feelings when not playing. Another symptom is

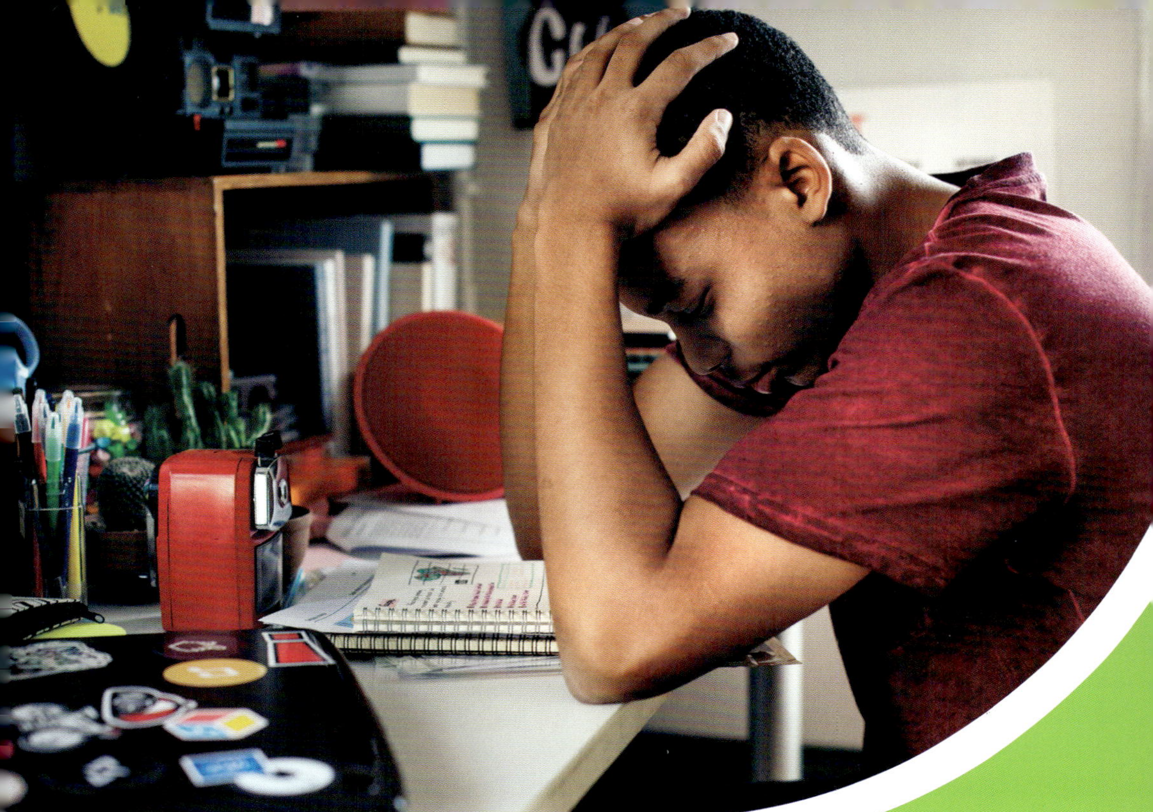

Video game addiction can make it tough to focus on other tasks.

spending an increasing amount of time

playing video games. Gamers may feel as

if they cannot control the amount of time

they spend playing. People may hide or

lie about their video game use. They may

lose interest in other hobbies. They may

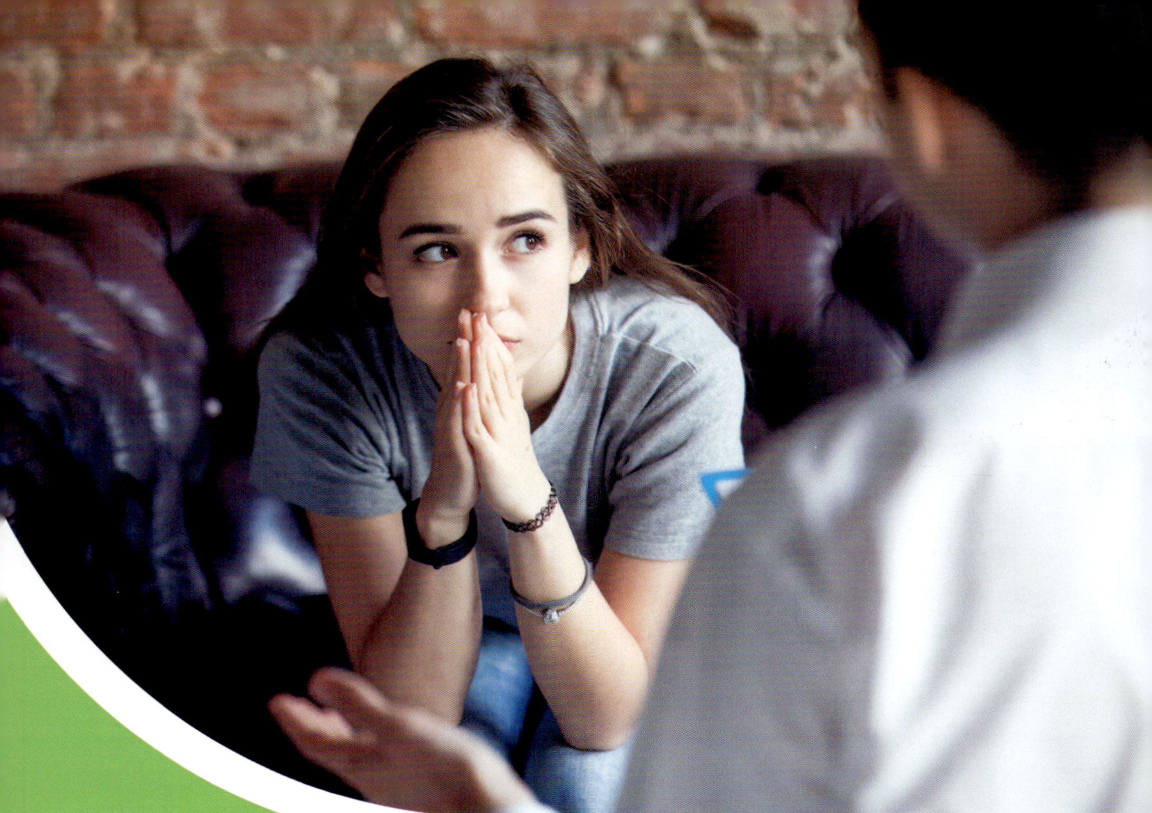

ignore the social strain video games cause.

Finally, their video game use may harm

their relationships at home or school. It

may affect their grades. Someone who

demonstrates five or more symptoms in a

year may be considered to have IGD.

However, the APA did not classify IGD as an official diagnosis in 2013. Instead, the APA identified gaming addiction as a condition needing more research. After five years of more research, the WHO recognized gaming addiction as a disorder in 2018. This recognition raised awareness of the condition. Increased awareness of gaming addiction provided opportunities for research and treatment.

GAMING DISORDER

Douglas A. Gentile is a psychology professor at Iowa State University.

He researches the effects of video games on the brain. Gentile has published many scientific papers on this topic. Some papers focus on video game addiction.

One of Gentile's papers is titled "Internet Gaming Disorder in Children and Adolescents." In it, Gentile states that "some heavy users of video games indeed develop **dysfunctional** symptoms that can result in severe . . . effects on functional and social areas of life."[3]

Researchers continue to debate whether gaming addiction is a disorder. Some experts believe the APA's gaming addiction

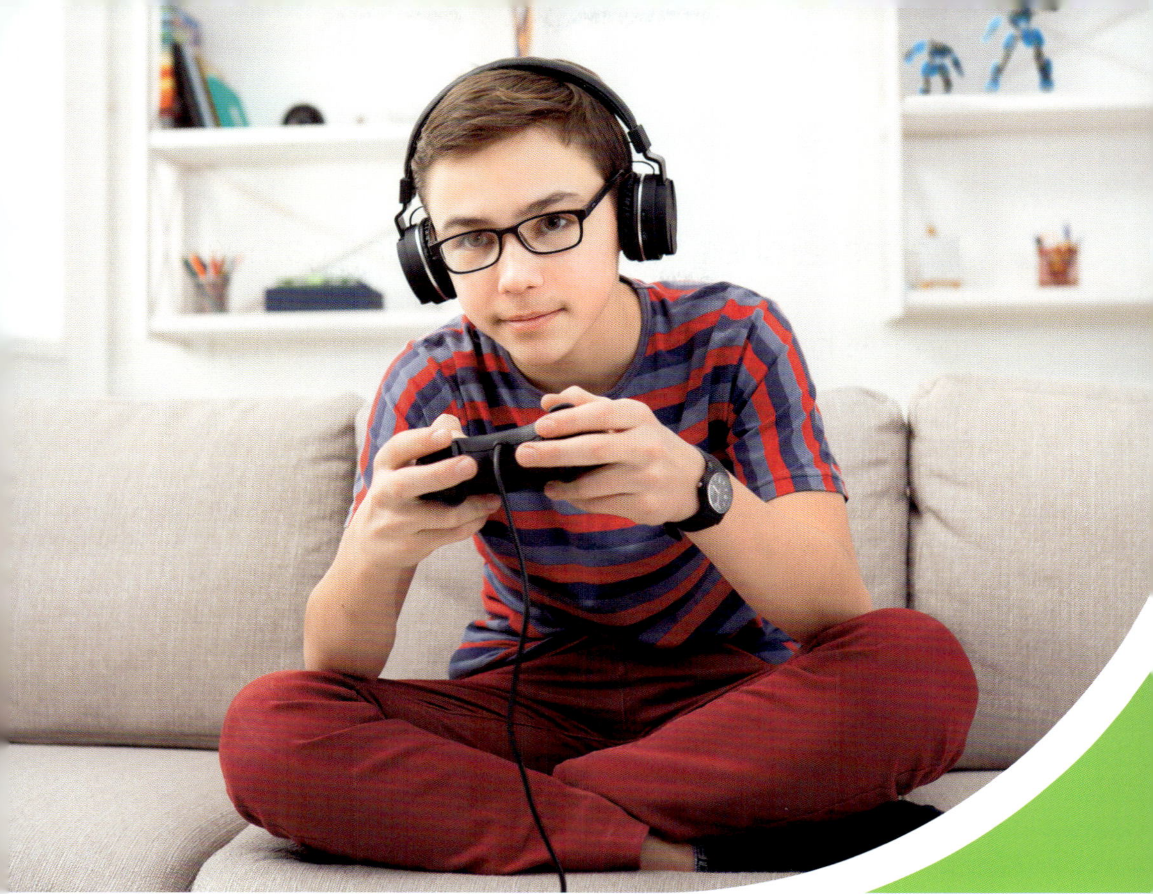

Not everyone who plays lots of video games is addicted.

symptoms are unclear. Certain behaviors

could also describe someone without a

gaming problem. For example, someone

could use video games to escape stressful

or sad real-life experiences. This does not

necessarily mean the person is addicted to video games. He or she could be gaming to cope with overwhelming feelings.

The Recovery Village is a **rehabilitation** facility in Florida. It helps people struggling with gaming and other addictions. "Individuals play video games for various reasons, whether it be for entertainment, competition, or as a coping mechanism for other conditions," its website states. "Video game addiction is also found to often co-occur with other conditions."[4] It is possible someone playing a lot of video games could be suffering from another

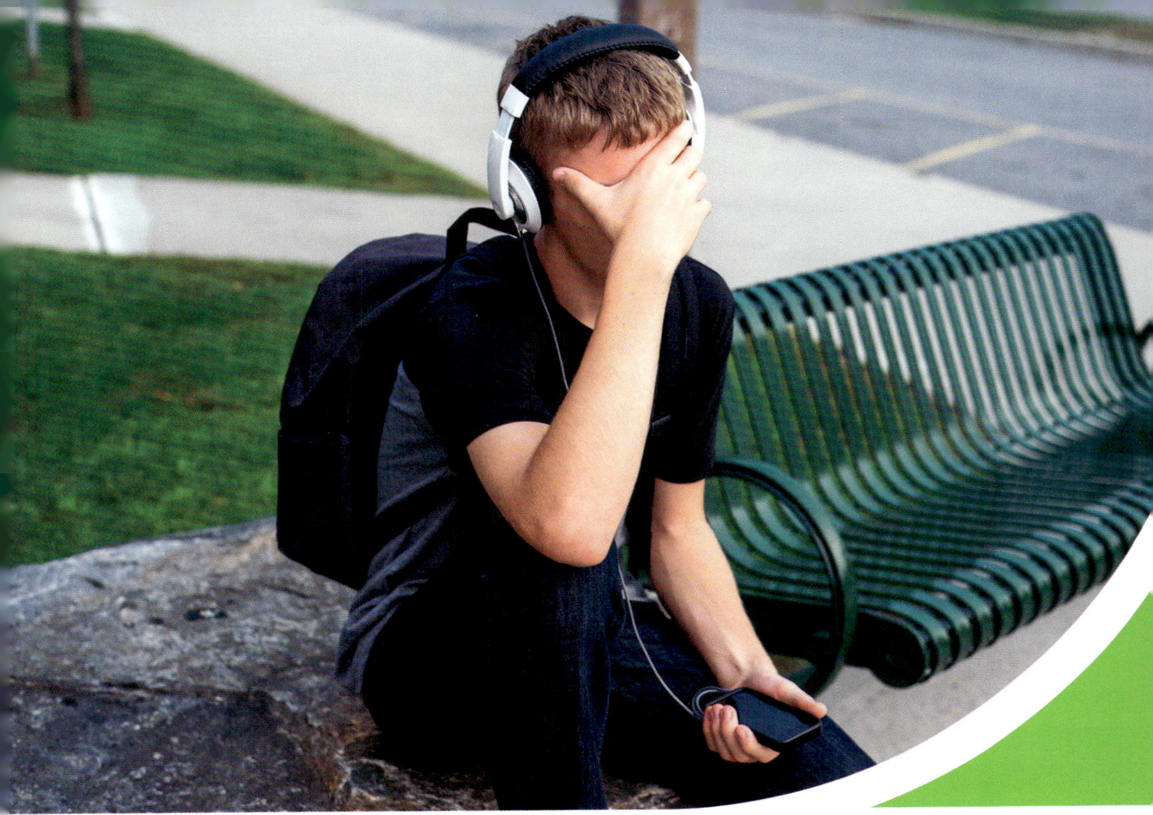

mental health disorder. Common mental health disorders include attention deficit disorder, anxiety, and **depression**.

Many experts agree the problem is not the number of hours spent gaming. The problem is the effect gaming has on a person's life. Gaming that causes people to neglect other parts of their lives is a problem. A person who continues to play games despite negative consequences might be addicted.

WHY ARE VIDEO GAMES ADDICTIVE?

Video games were invented more than fifty years ago. Since the invention of the first games, a lot has changed. Today, games are more portable and accessible than ever before. Gameplay has changed, too. Many modern video games are **immersive**. It is easy to lose track of time while playing.

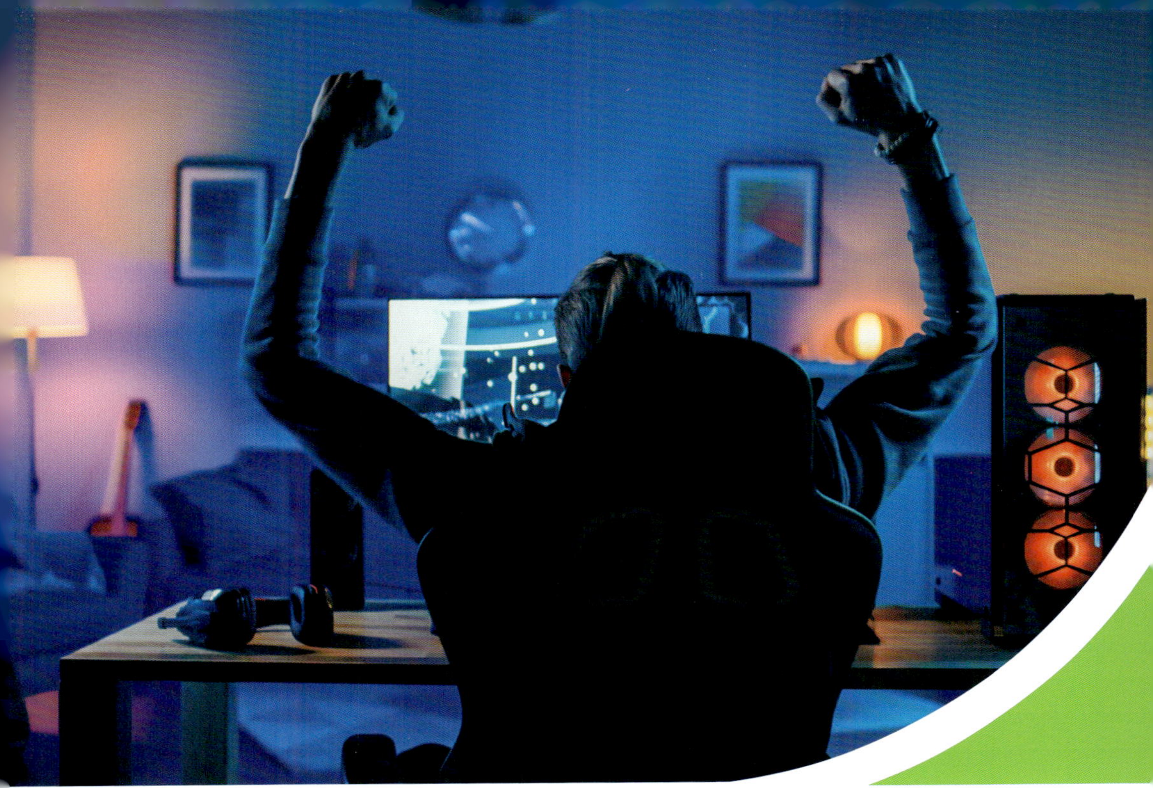

Beating an opponent or high score in a video game encourages a gamer to keep playing.

Certain types of games are designed

to encourage continued play more than

others. Massively multiplayer online

role-playing games (MMORPGs) are

popular. MMORPGs such as *World of*

Warcraft allow players to create unique

characters and explore imaginary worlds

with their friends. Battle royale games such

as *Fortnite* are designed to create a strong

desire to win. Each match starts with many

players. The last one standing is the winner.

Gamers might play over and over again to

get a victory.

These types of hooks are what make

games addictive. Hooks are features

included in games to keep people playing.

Hooks can be simple. Displaying high

scores is a simple hook. By displaying high

scores, a gamer always has a goal to beat.

Hooks can also be complex. Exploring a

COMMON HOOKS IN VIDEO GAMES

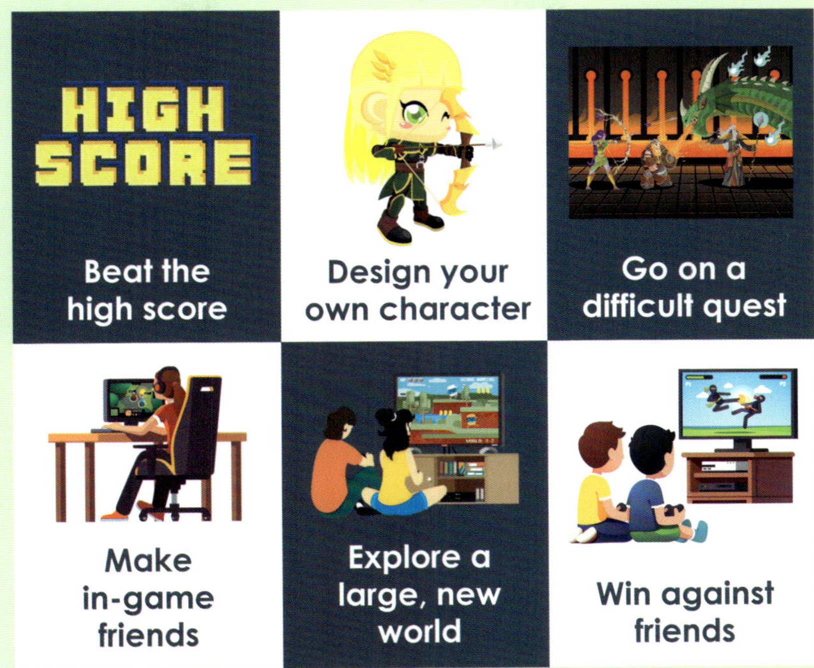

Source: "What Makes a Video Game Addictive?" Video Game Addiction, n.d. www.video-game-addiction.org.

Video game designers use several different types of hooks to keep players engaged.

unique world is a complex hook. In a unique

world, a gamer is eager to discover new

things. Both simple and complex hooks

encourage continued gameplay. These types of hooks only cost a player time.

However, other hooks cost real money. Loot boxes are one example. Loot boxes contain fun items for the game. These items might be just for looks. People might find a new style of armor or a dance animation for their character. But some items might improve gameplay. A person might find a better weapon or a power-up item. In most cases, users do not know what will be in a loot box when they buy it. As with gambling, people buy a loot box in hopes of obtaining a valuable item. Game addiction expert

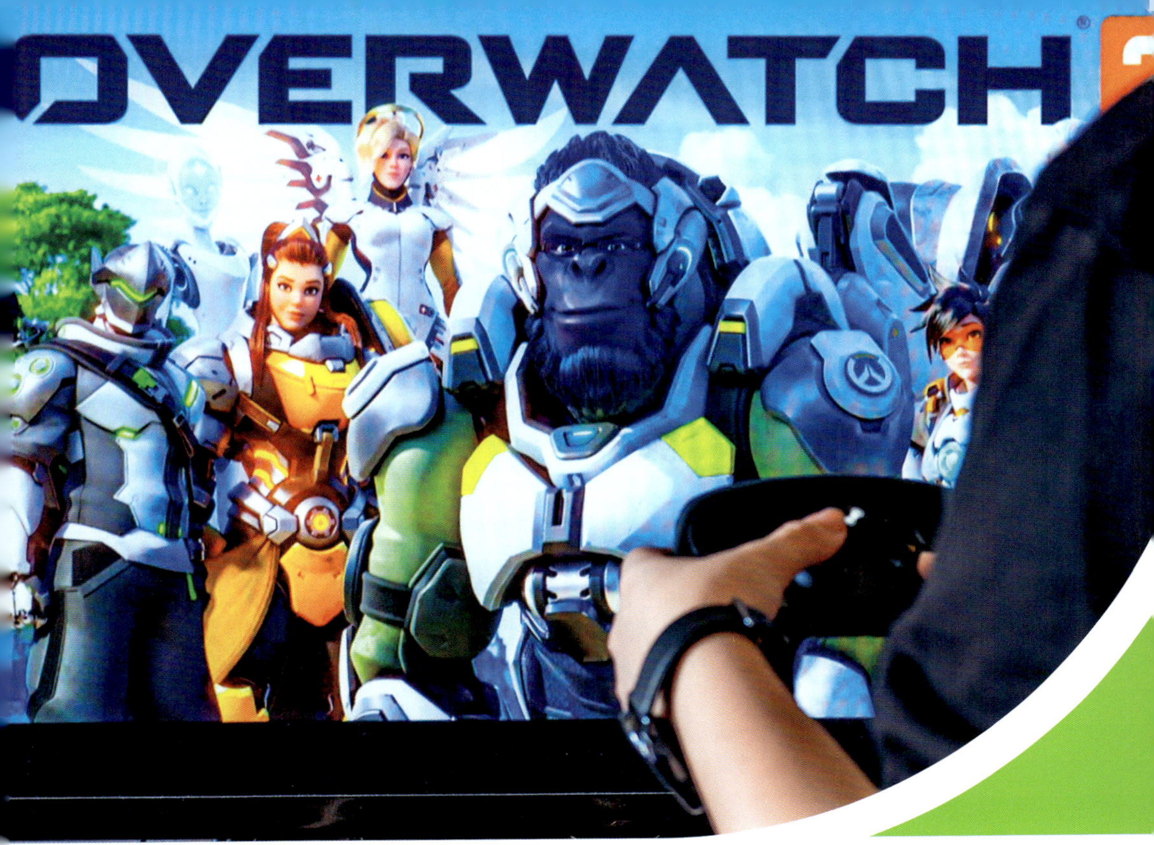

Many of the most popular video games sell loot boxes to players.

Cam Adair states, "Loot boxes appeal to individuals who are psychologically vulnerable and are open to the idea of gambling and buying loot crates."[5] People with gaming addiction might spend hundreds or thousands of dollars a year on

loot boxes and other in-game purchases.

Most hooks have one thing in common.

They stimulate the reward centers in

the brain. The brain's reward center is

a small cluster of nerve cells called the

nucleus accumbens. When a person does

something pleasurable, the brain releases a

substance called dopamine into the reward

center. This makes the person experience a

feeling of pleasure.

In people with gaming addiction,

these pleasures send the brain's reward

center into overdrive. The brain tries to

compensate by producing less dopamine. Over time, the brain adjusts to this stimulation. In terms of addiction, this is called tolerance. Normal things that used to be pleasurable no longer stimulate the reward center. To make up for this, people need to play more video games.

DOPAMINE

Dopamine is a brain chemical. It sends information between neurons in the brain. The brain releases dopamine when someone does something that is pleasurable. This could be eating a favorite food or playing a favorite game. Dopamine boosts people's mood and focuses their attention. It motivates them to continue the pleasurable behavior.

3
THE EFFECTS OF GAMING ADDICTION

Spending too much time gaming can have negative consequences. These consequences affect gamers as well as their friends and family. Elizabeth Hartney studies gaming addiction. She explains, "Video game addictions are similar to other addictions in terms of the amount of time spent playing, the strong emotional

attachment to the activity, and the patterns

of social difficulties experienced by gaming

addicts."[6]

People can enjoy video games in

moderation. But too much gaming takes

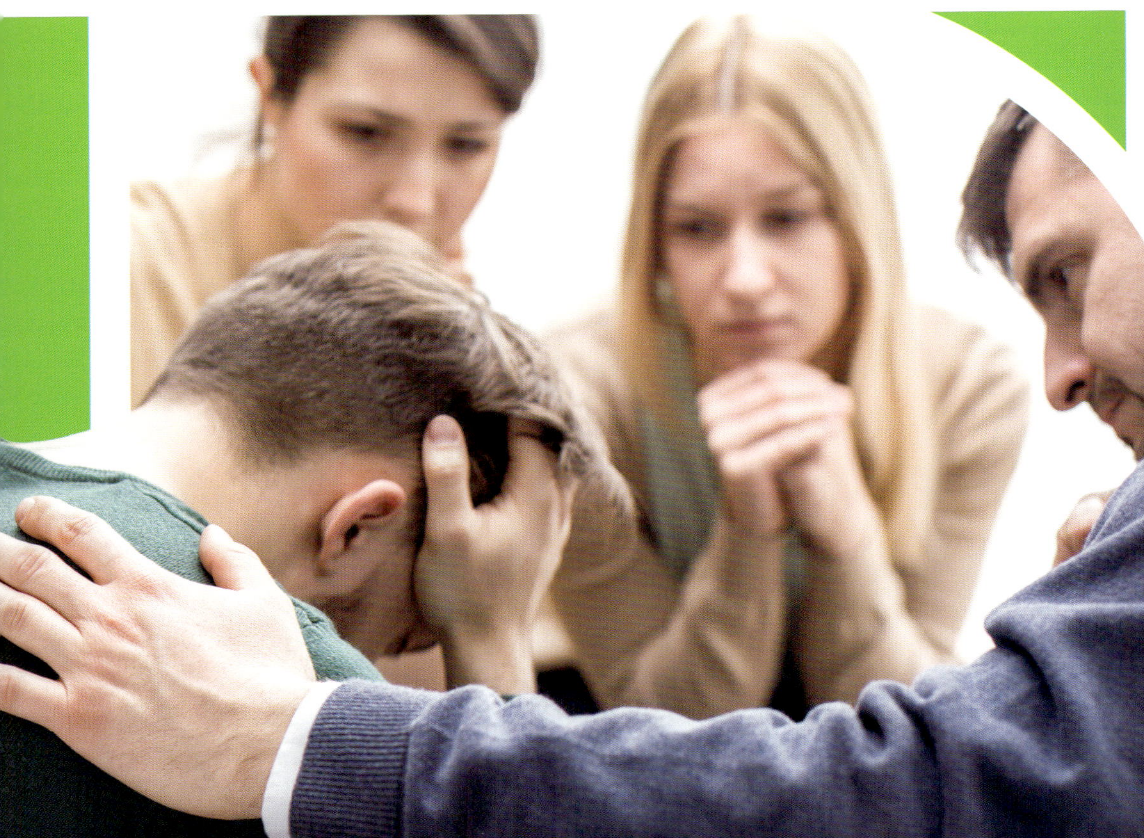

time away from other activities. Gaming
addiction can affect relationships as well as
mental and physical health.

PERSONAL CONSEQUENCES

Someone's physical and mental health
can suffer from gaming addiction. Some
of these effects are short-term. Others can
become long-term if the person's gaming
addiction continues.

Gaming addiction may cause a person to
skip meals or make unhealthy food choices.
This may make the person hungry in the
short term. However, poor eating habits

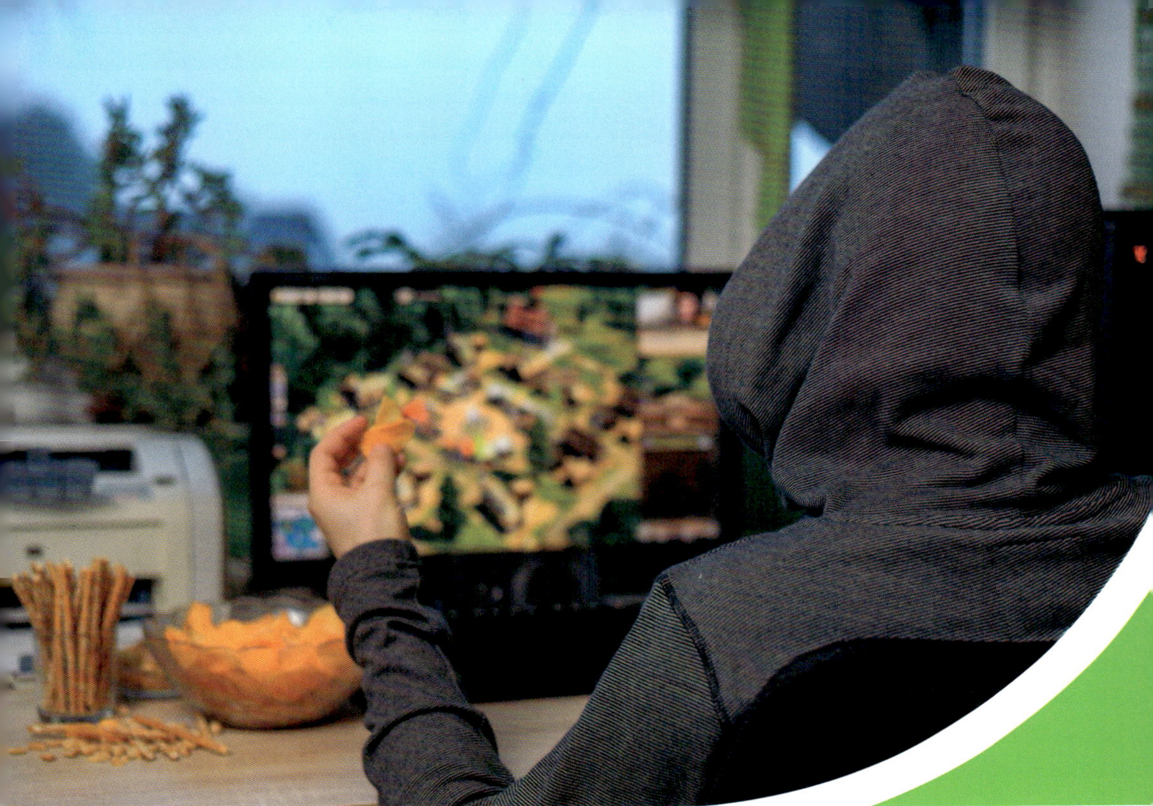

When video games become an obsession, someone may forget to eat a balanced diet.

can have long-term effects. Someone may experience weight loss or weight gain. The body might not get all the nutrients it needs. This can lead to other diet-related problems.

Spending lots of time gaming leaves little time for sleep. Short-term effects of not

sleeping include feeling drowsy or **fatigued**.
Other effects include doing poorly at school
and increased aggression. Over time, poor
sleep habits may cause difficulty falling or
staying asleep.

Gamers often spend a lot of time seated
and using a controller or keyboard. These
repetitive movements can cause problems.
Gamers might develop carpal tunnel
syndrome. This is a painful condition of the
hand. Gamers can also develop back pain
from sitting for hours.

Gaming addiction can cause money
problems, too. Games and consoles cost

money. However, in-game purchases are where most players spend a lot of money. Loot boxes and other purchases can add up quickly.

When gamers suffer physically and socially, their mental health suffers, too.

SHOULD LOOT BOXES BE REGULATED?

Loot boxes offer gamers a chance to win valuable in-game items. But winning is not guaranteed. Some people believe loot boxes are games of chance, as gambling is. They believe the government should limit who can purchase loot boxes. Loot boxes are considered gambling in Japan, Belgium, and the Netherlands. However, the United States has no laws regulating loot boxes.

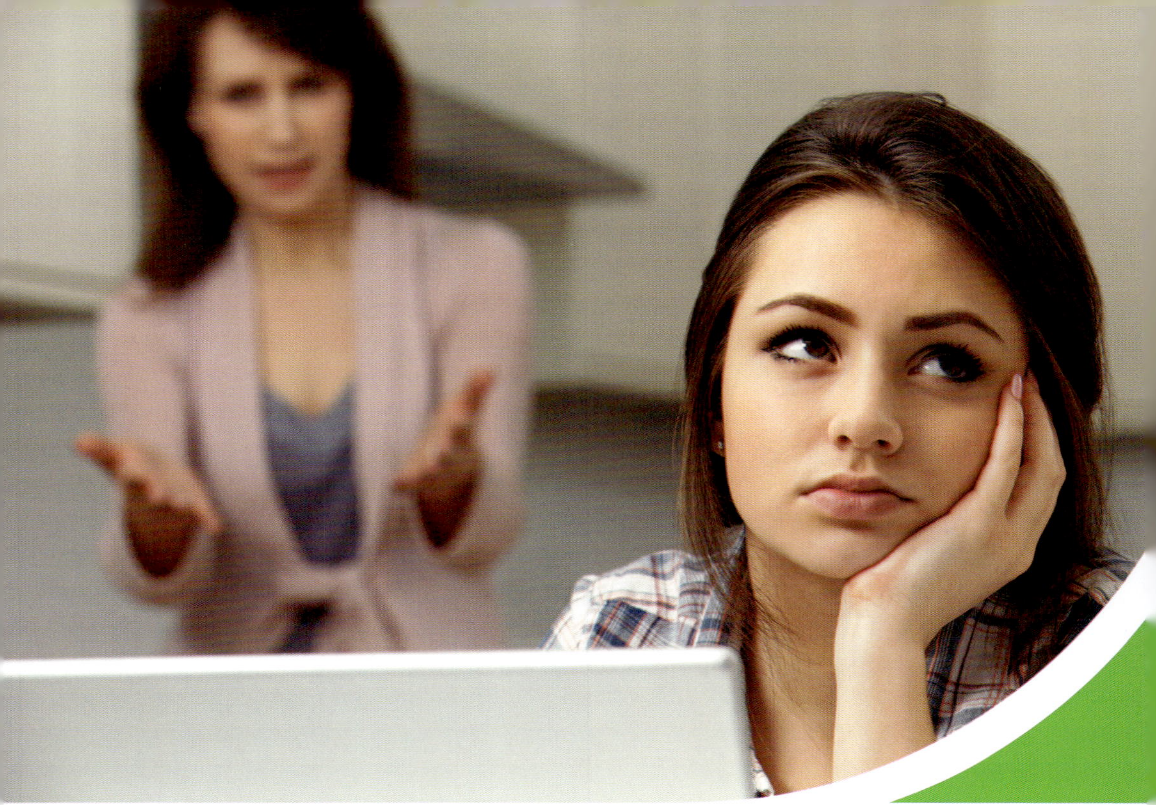

Too much gaming can lead to fights with parents.

A gamer can feel lonely and depressed. Gaming addiction causes people to feel anxious when they are not playing.

Gaming addiction can cause someone to do poorly in school. Gamers might fall asleep during class. They might skip school or not study. Experts also believe gaming

may reduce a person's attention span.

FAMILY AND FRIENDS

People close to someone addicted to

gaming can be affected in many ways.

Relationships with the person can fall apart.

The gamer might stop spending time with

friends and family to play more games.

Someone addicted to gaming might be

more angry than normal. This can cause the

gamer to treat friends and family differently.

The gamer might yell at family members or

even become violent.

4

TREATING GAMING ADDICTION

Without an official diagnosis from the APA, it is difficult for someone to get correctly diagnosed with IGD. This makes treatment for gaming addiction difficult.

Dr. Meredith E. Gansner states, "For gaming disorder, the lack of standardized research makes treatment decisions exceedingly challenging."[7] When the WHO

recognized gaming addiction as a disorder,

opportunities for research increased. More

treatment options will become available as

more researchers complete studies.

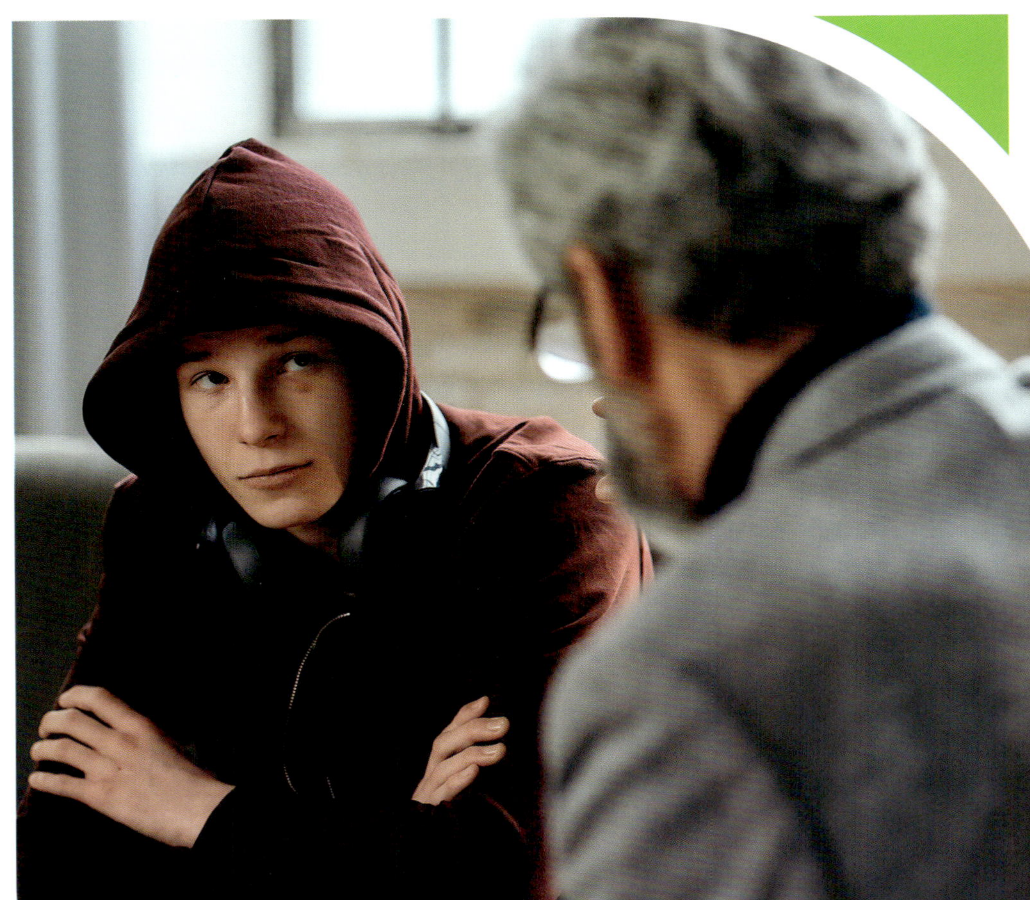

GETTING HELP

Gaming can be a problem even if a person is not diagnosed with gaming addiction. If gaming causes negative effects in a person's life, it is a problem. If gaming is a problem, there are ways to get help.

TREATING GAMING ADDICTION

Treatment for IGD gradually reduces the time someone spends gaming. It helps that person recognize his or her behavior as an addiction. Treatment uncovers triggers that cause the addiction. Then, it shows people how to avoid those triggers. Finally, treatment shows people how their behavior is harming themselves and loved ones.

A person can talk to a trusted adult, such as a parent or teacher. A gamer might seek professional support. It might be helpful to speak with a licensed therapist. Therapists with experience treating addictions can provide treatment options. A psychiatrist can help with addiction and other mental health concerns, too.

For physical problems, a gamer can go to a medical doctor. A medical doctor can provide treatment for physical health issues. The doctor might recommend working with a nutritionist. A nutritionist can help people develop healthier eating habits.

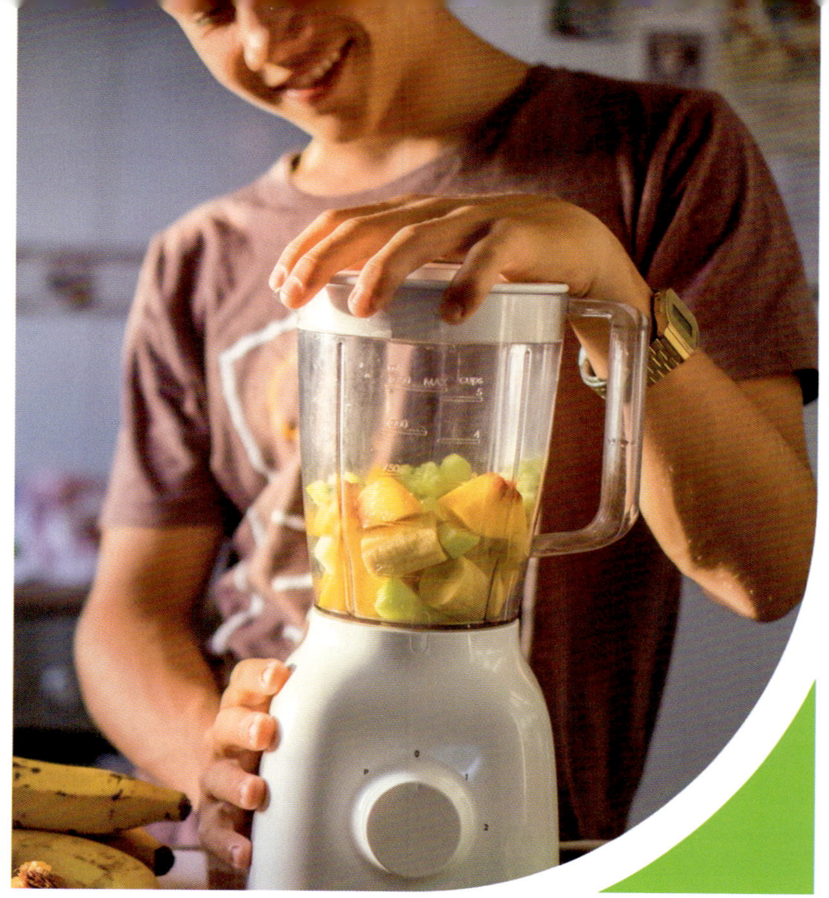

TREATMENT OPTIONS

There are resources available for gamers

dealing with addiction. One resource is

The Gaming Overload Workbook by Randy

Kulman. Kulman states, "The biggest

problem with video games is *not* that you can't learn all kinds of skills and knowledge, socialize with others, or have fun and challenge your brain—but that video games . . . sometimes don't leave enough time for other important things."[8]

Kulman's workbook takes a positive approach. It does not focus only on quitting gaming. Instead, it discusses other hobbies and interests. It asks readers to think about what they miss by only playing video games.

Additional treatment options involve help from other people. This could include joining

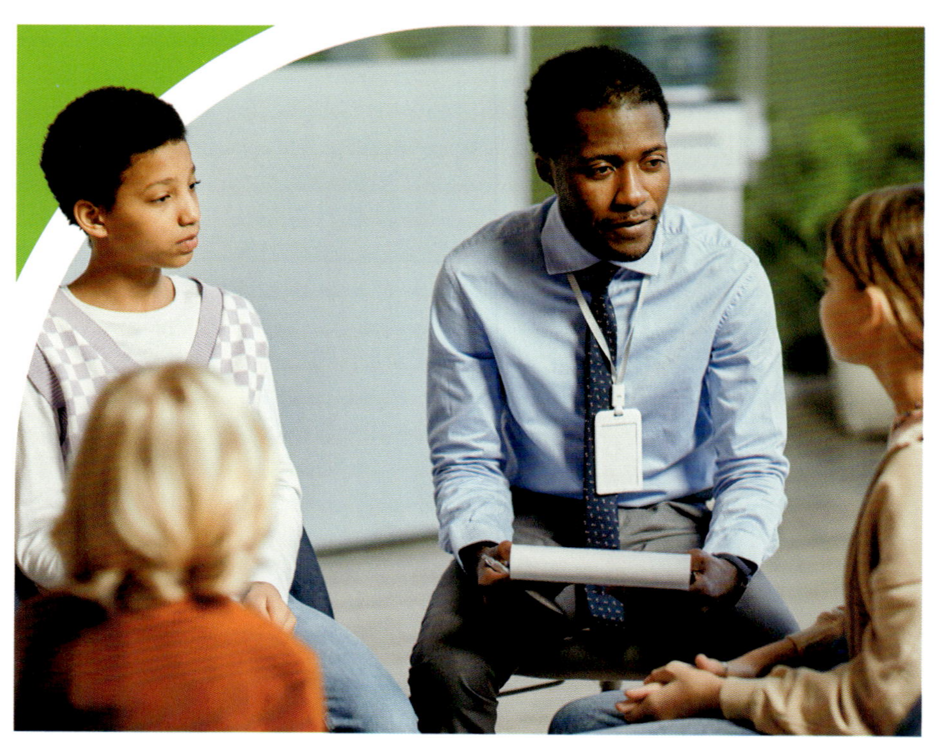

Group therapy can be a helpful treatment option for people with gaming addiction.

a group of people who are experiencing

gaming addiction. Group members offer

each other support.

Psychologists and psychiatrists can

provide treatment, too. These professionals

often use cognitive behavioral therapy

(CBT). This treatment helps people see how their thoughts, emotions, and actions are connected. By understanding this, people can change their behavior.

Extreme gaming is a behavior that can be changed. People who play games to relieve stress can learn other ways to relax. People who play games out of loneliness can seek out other social activities.

Video games are enjoyable. However, a small percentage of players will develop a gaming addiction. Researchers continue to study gaming addiction. More treatment options will become available in the future.

chronic

long-lasting

depression

a mental illness that causes feelings of sadness and loss of interest in enjoyable activities

dysfunctional

not functioning properly

fatigued

weary or exhausted

immersive

deeply absorbing and engaging

moderation

doing something in a non-extreme way

negative consequences

harmful results

neglect

give little attention to

rehabilitation

the process of recovering from an addiction

CHAPTER ONE: WHAT IS GAMING ADDICTION?

1. "Addictive Behaviours: Gaming Disorder," *Newsroom* (blog), *World Health Organization*, October 22, 2020. www.who.int.

2. Stanley Pierre-Louis, "ESA Leadership Desk: A Nation of Video Game Players," *News* (blog), *Entertainment Software Association*, July 13, 2021. www.theesa.com.

CHAPTER TWO: THE SCIENCE OF GAMING ADDICTION

3. Douglas A. Gentile et al., "Internet Gaming Disorder in Children and Adolescents," *Pediatrics* (2017) 140 (Supplement_2): S81–S85. https://doi.org/10.1542/peds.2016-1758H.

4. The Recovery Village, "Video Game Addiction Treatment," *The Recovery Village*, April 21, 2021. www.therecoveryvillage.com.

5. Cam Adair, "Loot Box Addiction: Dangers of Loot Boxes," *Game Quitters*, n.d. www.gamequitters.com.

CHAPTER THREE: THE EFFECTS OF GAMING ADDICTION

6. Elizabeth Hartney, "The Signs and Effects of Video Game Addiction," *VeryWell Mind*, May 16, 2020. www.verywellmind.com.

CHAPTER FOUR: TREATING GAMING ADDICTION

7. Meredith E. Gansner, "Gaming Addiction in ICD-11: Issues and Implications," *Psychiatric Times*, September 11, 2019. www.psychiatrictimes.com.

8. Randy Kulman, *The Gaming Overload Workbook: A Teen's Guide to Balancing Screen Time, Video Games, and Real Life*. Oakland, CA: New Harbinger Publications, 2020, p. 1.

FOR FURTHER RESEARCH

BOOKS

Tammy Gagne, *What Is Gaming Disorder?* San Diego, CA: ReferencePoint Press, 2021.

Randy Kulman, *The Gaming Overload Workbook: A Teen's Guide to Balancing Screen Time, Video Games, and Real Life.* Oakland, CA: New Harbinger Publications, 2020.

Bradley Steffens, *Addicted to Video Games.* San Diego, CA: ReferencePoint Press, 2019.

INTERNET SOURCES

Meredith E. Gansner, "Gaming Addiction in ICD-11: Issues and Implications," *Psychiatric Times*, September 11, 2019. www.psychiatrictimes.com.

Elizabeth Hartney, "The Signs and Effects of Video Game Addiction," *VeryWell Mind*, May 16, 2020. www.verywellmind.com.

The Recovery Village, "Video Game Addiction Statistics," *The Recovery Village*, April 21, 2021. www.therecoveryvillage.com.

WEBSITES

Game Quitters
https://gamequitters.com

Game Quitters is a resource for people experiencing addiction. It features programs for individuals and their families.

Internet Gaming
www.psychiatry.org/patients-families/internet-gaming

This website provides an overview of internet gaming disorder and the latest research into IGD.

Video Game Addiction
www.video-game-addiction.org

Video Game Addiction provides articles and resources for people experiencing symptoms of gaming addiction.

INDEX

IMAGE CREDITS

Cover: © Larisa Stefanjuk/Shutterstock Images

5: © Dean Drobot/Shutterstock Images

7: © Pixel Shot/Shutterstock Images

9: © Michael Kowalski/Shutterstock Images

11: © Jon Osumi/Shutterstock Images

13: © Sezer 66/Shutterstock Images

15: © Pixel Shot/Shutterstock Images

18: © Marc Bruxelle/Shutterstock Images

23: © Motortion Films/Shutterstock Images

25: © Dean Drobot/Shutterstock Images

27: © Raw Pixel/Shutterstock Images

28: © Fizkes/Shutterstock Images

31: © Prostock Studio/Shutterstock Images

33: © Moore Media/Shutterstock Images

35: © Gorodenkoff/Shutterstock Images

37 (top left): © Revel Stock Art/Shutterstock Images

37 (top middle): © Pzuh/Shutterstock Images

37 (top right): © Delcarmat/Shutterstock Images

37 (bottom left): © Iconic Bestiary/Shutterstock Images

37 (bottom middle): © Lucky Clover/Shutterstock Images

37 (bottom right): © Iconic Bestiary/Shutterstock Images

39: © Amlan Mathur/Alamy

43: © Photographee EU/Shutterstock Images

45: © Black Regis/Shutterstock Images

48: © Speed Kingz/Shutterstock Images

51: © Baza Production/Shutterstock Images

54: © Simona Pilolla 2/Shutterstock Images

56: © Seventy-Four/Shutterstock Images

ABOUT THE AUTHOR

Kizzi Roberts once joined the circus and traveled the country. Now her adventures are a little closer to home, where she spends her days writing and sometimes playing video games with her husband. She also enjoys sewing, Brazilian jiujitsu, and playing board games. She lives in the beautiful Ozarks with her family.